GMO and Glyphosate
ZEN

Roditch Roditch

Contents

Introduction

There is no greater danger to our peaceful and happy existence than GMO food that has been sprayed with glyphosate. Governments will not protect you from glyphosate or from poisonous food and water, 5G wireless networks, corrupt doctors, corrupt pharmaceutical companies, or pollution of all kinds. This is a required understanding to fully appreciate the sentiments in this book. Ask yourself? Which team are you on, the creators or the destroyers, and remind yourself why this is? It is important to understand that planet earth is a sensitive ecosystem, of which we are part, and we were never meant to dominate it because we don't have the heart and soul of the creator. There is no other way. Protect the earth or destroy it.

Just like 5G networks, there are a lot of studies that say glyphosate is harmless, as are GMO foods. When reading about their safety, most articles support the use of GMOs and glyphosate. Here is the problem: the huge power and influence companies like Monsanto (now Bayer) have over governments and the media creates the illusion that they are safe, when they are not. This is confusing and delays taking the necessary action to cease eating this kind of food and eat totally organic food instead.

Recently, people have sued Monsanto (and won) because they have acquired "Non-Hodgkin's lymphoma." Non-Hodgkin's lymphoma represents the fifth-leading type of cancer among both sexes, accounting for 4-5% of new cancer cases and 3% of cancer deaths. The incidence rates in the US doubled between 1970 and 1990. Interestingly, this is when Monsanto discovered glyphosate and created Roundup. John E. Franz (born December 21, 1929) is an organic chemist who discovered the herbicide glyphosate while working at Monsanto Company in 1970. The chemical became the active ingredient in Roundup, a broad-spectrum, post-emergence herbicide.

The most characteristic symptom of non-Hodgkin's lymphoma is a painless swelling in a lymph node, usually observed in the neck, armpit, or groin. Most patients will receive chemotherapy with or without radiotherapy.

The evidence is clear enough: glyphosate is poisonous. For courts to award millions of dollars to people who have developed cancer from using Roundup, there has to be some evidence.

There are so many ways we can become seriously ill: contaminated water, air pollution, stress, non-organic food, using industrial and household chemicals, smoking, drinking alcohol, junk food, lacking sunlight, a lack of fruit, vegetables, and herbs, etc. We are being bombarded by disease-causing substances every minute because industries and governments want our money.

There is no doubt in my mind that as we shift away from the natural (non-industrialized) foods that we used to eat, we are much more susceptible to diseases like cancer and diabetes. This small book introduces the conversation that we all need to have as families, partners, co-workers, and individuals: we cannot live long and healthy lives if we continue to believe everything we read about health in the media. We must remember how the earth was created with our every need supported and supplied for, and it was created perfectly. With the onset of merchants who discovered they could take our money out of our pockets legally, core values of honesty, integrity, and wisdom have been replaced by making a "quick buck."

To survive the merchants, we have to take affirmative action: eat only organic food, drink only pure water, breathe only pure air, and have plenty of debt-free time to exercise and commune with nature. This is quite easy once you decide that organic food tastes better, keeps better, has many more vitamins and minerals, and is poison-free. that all these benefits far outweigh the extra cost of purchasing organic food. There are also huge savings to be had. Organic food will give you more time, because when you are healthy, you and your children will hardly ever get sick. You will never have to see the doctor and will probably live a long and happy life.

A family who all became sick and then cured themselves with an organic diet clearly outlines the dangers of having your immune system compromised by GMO and glyphosate foods. All four of them developed different, serious diseases that were completely cured by eating 100% organic foods. The causes of most diseases are shrouded in mystery because governments and doctors don't care. Once you understand this truth, your life will change completely. Never forget, doctors need our money, and so does President Trump if he wants to fly around the world in a big blue jet, we all paid for.

After doing research, it became clear to me that good health and longevity come from reducing (cutting out) toxins and increasing natural nutrients (vitamins, minerals, enzymes, and fats). GMO food and glyphosate add to the already numerous poisons we consume every day, which tips us into very dangerous territory. Organic food, on the other hand, tends to be very healthy. When you consume organic food, you are cutting out all the poisons and increasing your intake of natural nutrients—considerably.

Glyphosate

Glyphosate is a chemical originally used to clean out industrial pipes. A chemist at Monsanto discovered it killed weeds, and Monsanto started manufacturing Roundup in the 1970s. Glyphosate is one of the most heavily studied chemicals in history. Glyphosate is derived from an amino acid, glycine. It acts by suppressing an essential biochemical mechanism commonly found in plants but not in animals. It is designed to specifically inhibit an enzymatic pathway required for protein synthesis—and thereby, growth—unique to plants.

According to the Extension Toxicology Network, a joint university pesticide information project, glyphosate is non-volatile, minimizing exposure through inhalation, and undergoes little metabolism in the human body. If accidentally consumed, glyphosate is excreted mostly unchanged in feces and urine, so it doesn't stay in the body and accumulate. Glyphosate, commonly known by its original trade name Roundup (manufactured by Monsanto), is the world's most widely used herbicide (weedkiller). Glyphosate-based herbicides are manufactured by many companies in many countries.

Glyphosate is used on many crops to control weeds, including about 80% of genetically modified (GM) crops. Seeds are modified to be resistant to glyphosate so that when the herbicide is used, it kills only the weeds around the crops. It is also sprayed on many crops, including cereals such as wheat and oats, as a pre-harvest desiccant. This encourages the crops to dry quickly and evenly, allowing for earlier harvesting.

Subchronic and chronic tests with glyphosate have been conducted with rats, dogs, mice, and rabbits in studies lasting from 21 days to two years. With a few exceptions, there were no treatment-related gross (easily observable) or cellular changes. In a chronic feeding study with rats, no toxic effects were observed in rats given doses as high as 31 mg/kg/day, the highest dose tested. No toxic effects were observed in a chronic feeding study with dogs fed up to 500 mg/kg/day, the highest dose tested. Mice fed glyphosate for 90 days exhibited reduced body weight gains. The lifetime administration of very high amounts of glyphosate produced only a slight reduction in body weight and some microscopic liver and kidney changes. Blood chemistry, cellular components, and organ function were not affected even at the highest doses. "Hens fed massive amounts over three days and again 21 days later showed no nerve-related effects.

These results of research from Cornell University are impossible to believe after people are now being awarded millions of dollars in damages because there is clear evidence glyphosate causes cancer.

Narrative is becoming an important and popular way to describe the way governments and chemical companies bamboozle everyone with their lies, like in this example from a university.

There is also confusion about the safety of glyphosate in research because it is more dangerous when mixed as a formulation than by itself. Germany's authorities found in 2015 that the surfactant polyethoxylated tallowamine (POE tallowamine) contributed a large amount of toxicity to the herbicides it was used in, such as Roundup. This led to an EU-wide reassessment by the EFSA, which concluded that "a likely explanation for the poisoning occurrences observed in humans is that they are mostly driven by the POE-tallowamine component of the formulation." The E.U. subsequently decided to ban the use of the co-formulant.

There are other chemicals used when growing major crops that contribute to the toxicity of our food, like imidacloprid, which is used to coat seeds so they won't be eaten by birds. Roundup, a glyphosate-based, organophosphate weedkiller, is one of, if not the most widely used pesticide in the world. A formal review of glyphosate by the EPA and the Agency for Toxic Substances and Disease Registry (ATSDR) released this month found some statistically significant links to certain cancers, such as non-Hodgkin's lymphoma.

Farmworkers face significantly higher exposure than the general population. Pesticides have been linked to a list of long-term health issues, including prostate, lung, thyroid, and bone marrow cancer; diabetes; Parkinson's disease; asthma; and macular degeneration, according to the Agricultural Health Study, a government-funded research study that has monitored nearly 90,000 farmers and their spouses since the early 1990s. Acute pesticide poisoning may cause, along with short-term effects, long-term neurological damage, an EPA manual for healthcare providers warns.

Organophosphate (OP) pesticides, which include glyphosate and chlorpyrifos, have been targeted by some researchers as especially harmful. In a 2018 meta-review of OP health studies, University of California researchers discovered "compelling evidence" that prenatal exposure increases the risk of neurodevelopmental disorders and cognitive and behavioral deficits. Those researchers urged governments around the world to phase out the chemicals entirely. As of April, the EPA is under court order to decide whether to ban chlorpyrifos, which the agency found in 2017 to exceed safety standards for pesticide residue in food and water.

GMO Food

The combination of Glyphosate and GMO food creates chronic diseases in people of all ages: autism, neuropathy, cancer, asthma, allergies, development disorders, and rashes. The only way to get better is to eat pure organic food.

Many scientists don't agree with Bayer's narrative of safety, which influences most media coverage. They say it is the most radical change in our food supply and poses the greatest risks to our health. To create GMOs, scientists either take genes from one species and artificially force them into the DNA of another species or alter genes within the same species. This is not hybridization that uses the plant's own natural reproductive system; these are artificial techniques done in a laboratory; the process itself causes massive collateral damage to the DNA, which can increase toxins, allergens, new diseases, and nutritional problems. GMO soy, for example, has up to seven times the amount of an allergen.

One type of GMO corn contains a totally new allergen; another has more than 200 altered proteins and metabolites, including those linked to allergic reactions and cancer. These types of unpredicted changes may help explain why lab animals fed GMOs suffer from a variety of health issues. There are genetically engineered soy, corn, sugar beets, cotton, canola, and alfalfa—these are the six main GMOs. There's also papaya from China or Hawaii, as well as some zucchini or yellow squash, and a small amount of genetically engineered potatoes and apples just came onto the market. When you remove these foods, you're taking the biggest burden off your body because if those foods are removed, you've eliminated so much of the dysfunction. The more organic, non-GMO foods you eat, the healthier you will be. not days, but weeks or months to see the changes.

The primary reason Monsanto created genetically engineered crops is to allow that crop to be sprayed with their chemical herbicides, the most widely used is Monsanto's Roundup herbicide which would normally kill the weeds and the crops but their genetically engineered and designed seeds sprayed with Roundup and survive. These crops are called Roundup Ready. Over 80% of all GMO crops worldwide are Monsanto's Roundup Ready varieties.

Roundup was originally patented as an industrial cleaner to clean boilers and pipes. It grabs on to the minerals and strips the buildup inside the pipes. One day, when the residue spilled on the ground, it wiped out all the plants, so Monsanto bought glyphosate and patented it as an herbicide. It takes out metals, and that's not a good thing for all of us; we need to be able to absorb certain minerals into our bodies. They also damage the gut microbiome, which, as we now understand, affects human health and even brain health. We call the bacteria and the other organisms the "human microbiome." The cutting edge of medicine right now is about the organisms that live from your mouth to your behind. The trillions of bacteria in your body control many aspects of your health, including your immunity and the metabolism of vitamins. It's the first line of defense for detoxification. Your set point for inflammation, for example, is mediated by your gut bacteria. They are your buddies; you must love your microbiome; they make the very chemistry that rules your brain—the brain chemistry that makes you happy or sad.

When roundup first came out on the market, we were told that it wouldn't affect human health because humans don't have the "chicken mate pathway," which is a pathway that plants have, and that's where roundup affects plants. We don't have this pathway, but our gut bacteria do, and without our gut bacteria, we can't produce the compounds from certain amino acids to make these other chemicals that we need to run our entire body: things like tyrosine and tryptophan.

Tyrosine makes dopamine, and tryptophan makes serotonin; both are considered feel-good chemicals. More than 90% of the serotonin in the body is actually manufactured in the gut, so when you unleash a chemical like glyphosate that damages the gut bacteria, there is hell to pay. There are consequences that we are just beginning to understand that are very real. We know what glyphosate does; it's been patented as an antibiotic. The last thing we want to bring into the body is an antibiotic, particularly on food, because our microbiome, or our bacteria, is really our number one defense; it kills the beneficial gut bacteria. The probiotics we normally pay for, like Lactobacillus, don't kill the nasty stuff like pathogenic E. coli, Salmonella, and botulism, which can overgrow in our gut. Sometimes pathogenic gut bacteria lead to inflammation in the brain, which can lead to behavioral issues and very high levels of fungus. The same fungus that is present in children with autism is also Clostridium difficile. This can also cause leaky gut, which is an infection of the intestines.

Autism, Alzheimer's, Parkinson's, and multiple sclerosis are inflammatory diseases of the brain, and it's the bacteria in the gut that regulate inflammation, and these are the bacteria that are damaged when they are exposed to glyphosate.

After switching to non-GMO diets, you will have significant improvements in more than 20 other health issues, including energy level, weight loss, brain fog, allergies, anxiety, depression, memory, pain, insomnia, hormone problems, gluten sensitivity, diabetes, and skin disorders.

There are also corn and cotton plants engineered to produce their own toxic insecticide called Bt toxin. The BT-toxin breaks open little holes in the walls of the insect's gut and kills it. Both BT toxin and roundup can create a leaky gut. Permeable gut holes in the walls of our intestines compromise the function of what are called the mitochondria. People experience brain fog, and glyphosate does that. Your mitochondria are like little furnaces in each of your cells, and that's really where your energy is made—the energy that just keeps you alive. It's not a process that's passive to stay alive; it's an active process.

Roundup may affect many of our hormones, including the balance of testosterone and estrogen. The World Health Organization has now classified glyphosate as a probable human carcinogen, which is earth-shaking. According to the World Health Organization, glyphosate causes cancer in animals. The experiments that they did clearly showed that glyphosate causes several different types of lung cancer as well as interstitial destruction of the cells of the lungs, which would lead to COPD and asthma-like conditions. More than 400 scientists conclude GMOs are not the solution to world hunger. Ultra-low doses of Roundup caused non-alcoholic fatty liver disease in rats. One-quarter of Americans suffer from this liver disease, which is directly linked to obesity, diabetes, and heart disease.

To avoid GMOs and toxic pesticides you need to buy food that is labelled organic.

Antibiotic Resistance

A new study finds that bacteria develop antibiotic resistance up to 100,000 times faster when exposed to the world's most widely used herbicides, Roundup (Glyphosate) and Kamba (Dicamba), and antibiotics than when not exposed to the herbicide.

This study adds to a growing body of evidence that herbicides used on a mass industrial scale but not intended to be antibiotics can have profound effects on bacteria, with potentially negative implications for medicine's ability to treat infectious diseases caused by bacteria.

The combination of chemicals to which bacteria are exposed in the modern environment should be addressed alongside antibiotic use if we are to preserve antibiotics in the long-term.

An important finding of the new study was that even in cases where the herbicides increased the toxicity of antibiotics, they also significantly increased the rate of antibiotic resistance, which the study's authors say could be contributing to the greater use of antibiotics in both agriculture and medicine.

Previously, these researchers found that exposure to the herbicide products Roundup, Kamba, and 2,4-D or the active ingredients alone most often increased resistance but sometimes increased the susceptibility of potential human pathogens such as Salmonella enterica and Escherichia coli depending on the antibiotic.

When a drug or other chemical makes antibiotics more potent, that should be a good thing. But it also makes the antibiotic more effective at promoting resistance when it is at lower concentrations, as we more often find it in the environment.

BT Toxins

Bacillus thuringiensis (often referred to as simply "Bt") is a common, naturally occurring bacterium found in soils and on plant leaves worldwide. First discovered in 1901 in Japan, Bt has revolutionized how we stop insects from eating our crops. For over fifty years, Bt has been applied directly to a variety of agricultural crops and plants in home gardens as a living pesticide to control insect pests.

The secret to Bt's success is a family of proteins that these bacteria produce that specifically target insect digestive tracts. These proteins are shaped like crystals, so they are commonly called "Crystalline toxins" or "Cry toxins." These Cry toxins remain inactive until consumed by an insect. Once digested, the protein is activated and then binds to specific receptors in insect guts. Once bound, the Cry toxins pierce holes in the insect's gut, ultimately causing the contents to leak and the insect to starve. Importantly, humans do not have the same receptors or gut conditions as insects, which means Cry toxins pass through us with no effect. Studies show that humans digest Cry toxins like any other protein that would be ingested when eating foods like meat, beans, leafy greens, or tofu.

Many types of crytotoxins exist with varying specificity for different insects (primarily moths and butterflies, beetles, and flies). The diverse CR toxins can be mixed and matched to control several pests at once.

The chief benefit claimed for GMO insecticidal Bt crops is that, unlike conventional pesticides, their toxicity is limited to a few insect species. But a new peer-reviewed analysis systematically compares GMO and natural Bt proteins and shows that many of the elements contributing to this narrow toxicity have been removed by GMO developers in the process of inserting Bt toxins into crops. Thus, developers have made GMO insecticides that, in the words of one Monsanto patent, are "super toxins."

Biome and the Immune system

Our bodies harbor a huge array of microorganisms. While bacteria are the biggest players, we also host single-celled organisms known as archaea, as well as fungi, viruses, and other microbes—including viruses that attack bacteria. Together, these are dubbed the human microbiota. Your body's microbiome is all the genes your microbiota contains; however, colloquially, the two terms are often used interchangeably. Key roles of our microbes include programming the immune system, providing nutrients for our cells, and preventing colonization by harmful bacteria and viruses.

Human cells don't just contain chromosomes; they also carry DNA within our cellular powerhouses, the mitochondria, which are evolutionary descendants of bacteria. Our genome also contains stretches of genetic material called transposons that, at least in some cases, are thought to have been introduced long ago by viruses. "I prefer to define a human in evolutionary terms, and if we do this, then mitochondria are parts of a human, and so are transposons." Variability in the gut microbiome helps explain why people respond differently to the same foods. Whether tomatoes are good or bad for you, whether rice is good for you or worse for you than ice cream, and so on, is explained by your microbiome.

When GMO foods and glyphosate destroy the balance of healthy bacteria in your digestive system (directly from their unhealthy nature and from the decimation of your "good bacteria"), you will suffer typical digestive problems like diarrhea, stomach aches, and malnutrition. More importantly, your immune system is connected to your biome (the world of microbes in and on us). Once the healthy bacteria are compromised, your immune system is substantially weakened. Once weakened, you are susceptible to every disease in the doctor's manual.

Whether you have a serious health condition already or not, the four most important things you have to urgently do are: Eat only organic food and water; rebuild your biome using probiotics and prebiotics (kefir, kimchi, sauerkraut, garlic, onion, yoghurt). Make a general herbal mixture you can take every day (ginger, turmeric, moringa, Andrographis, mango leaves, and astragalus) and drink fresh organic fruit and vegetable juices (carrot, celery, apple, etc.). There are so many good herbs you can take either powdered or fresh that will help keep your immune and biomedical systems strong and healthy. You can buy a herb book and research on the internet all the herbs available around the world that can keep you healthy for 100 years; it's up to you, as always. You have an incredible power to manage your health if you take these simple steps.

Every time you take antibiotics, they kill good and bad bacteria. This often causes upset stomachs, a weakened immune system, and lots of confusion. Doctors never tell you to take probiotics for one month after taking a course of antibiotics. This is extremely unprofessional and dangerous. You should never take antibiotics for the flu unless it has become pneumonia. Antibiotics reduce your immunity and increase the flu's power. With a weakened immune system, the flu may return every few months because your immune system lacks the power to overpower the flu and make it submit. And, often with bacterial infections, natural things like garlic, Manuka honey, and ginger do a better job anyway. When you eat glyphosate-infused and GMO foods AND take antibiotics, you seriously need to take as many probiotics as you can, both supplements and natural ones.

Probiotics

As already discussed probiotics rebalance and support your intestinal flora (microbial biome). Glyphosate, GMO, and antibiotics destroy it.

Probiotics are a form of good bacteria found in your gut that are responsible for everything from nutrient absorption to immune health. Not only are probiotics essential for digestion, but did you know there are hundreds of other health benefits of consuming probiotic-rich foods that you might not be aware of? According to a review published in the journal ISRN Nutrition, probiotics could also help lower cholesterol, protect against allergies, aid in cancer prevention, and more.

In most cases, getting more probiotics in your diet doesn't require you to buy expensive pills, powders, or supplements. In fact, there are a number of probiotic foods out there that are delicious, versatile, and easy to enjoy as part of a healthy, well-rounded diet. Seven Types of "Friendly" Bacteria: Lactobacillus acidophilus, Lactobacillus bulgarius, Lactobacillus reuteri, Streptococcus thermophiles, Saccharomyces boulardii, Bifidobacterium bifidum, and Bacillus subtilis.

Here are some good natural probiotic foods you can eat every day.

Kefir is similar to yogurt, but because it is fermented with yeast and there are more bacteria.

Sauerkraut made from fermented cabbage and other probiotic vegetables. Sauerkraut is not diverse in probiotics but is high in organic acids.

Kombucha is an effervescent fermentation of black tea that is started by using a SCOBY.

Coconut Kefir made by fermenting the juice of young coconuts with kefir grains.

Yogurt is possibly the most popular probiotic food.

Kvass is made using probiotic fruits and beets along with other root vegetables like carrots.

Raw Cheese as goat's milk, sheep's milk and A2 cows. Soft cheeses are particularly high in probiotics.

Apple cider vinegar is a good source of probiotics.

Salted Gherkin Pickles homemade are the best.

Olives cured in brine.

Tempeh from Indonesia. This fermented soybean product is another source of probiotics.

Miso It is created by fermenting soybean, barley, or brown rice with koji.

Buttermilk, also sometimes called cultured buttermilk, is a fermented dairy drink that is made from the liquid that is leftover after churning butter.

Water kefir is made by adding kefir grains to sugar water, resulting in a fermented, fizzy beverage that is jam-packed with probiotics.

Raw milk. Raw cow's milk, goat's milk, sheep's milk and A2 aged cheeses are particularly high in probiotics.

Kimchi is a cousin to sauerkraut and is the Korean take on cultured veggies.

Tua Nao or **Natto** are fermented soybeans made in Thailand and Japan.

What we know so far

As Doctor Keith Scott-Mumby has said, when our bodies are overloaded with "bad stuff," disease will happen. He says we must keep the toxic load to a minimum to stay healthy. We know that when corporations working side by side with governments want to make large profits, they will create a false narrative about the health of their products, including GMOs, glyphosate, 5G networks, and factory-farmed food. So, you must dig a bit deeper for the truth. If you are still not sure about the safety of eating industrial food, all you must do is accept that organic food is much better for you. We also know that GMOs and glyphosate cause cancer and destroy our immune systems, leaving us prey to many kinds of diseases at any age. We know that to stay healthy and cure chronic diseases, we must eat and drink only organic food, take fresh or powdered herbs, and take the required action to change our lifestyle. Finally, we know that junk foods are either comfort foods or fast, convenient foods.

The desire for these foods begins in childhood, and for most of the population, this desire never changes. But, unfortunately, as we get older, we reap what we have sown. For the joy of staying a child and eating all that salty and sweet food, we will get sick in our 50s and pay the price with more frequent trips to the doctor and hospital. There is nothing difficult about eating healthy, organic food. Organic vegetables and fruit keep much longer, taste much better, and are your guarantee against early life retirement. I think of junk food (which includes all normal junk food and all supermarket food as well) the same as smoking and drinking: they are all poisonous, and one day we will pay dearly—with your life.

This book is simple advice, based on evidence, about the need to change your eating habits so you will have a long and happy life. It is about corporations and governments controlling the food we eat for profit—not just food but many aspects of our lives like health care, pharmaceuticals, and the internet.

We all have free will, even if we choose never to use it (based on fear and ignorance). It is important to wake up every morning and remind yourself that you have all the power over your own life you need as long as you exercise it.

Many people who abuse their bodies with tobacco, alcohol, and junk food are living a fantasy inside their own minds. It is important to understand that our mind is a tool that can be controlled for good or the opposite; it can control us with negative thoughts emanating from our subconscious. The mind left uncontrolled (Buddhists control it with meditation) builds a power of its own, like a virus running around our mindless lives: death by uncontrolled thought in a thousand strokes or less.

The world is changing rapidly. People are making billions like we once made millions. Soon, it will be trillions instead of billions. The oligarchs with this kind of money will rule the world, and we will be their slaves. This time is now, and it's getting worse by the day. While we find our way in this new world, we need to be healthy and debt-free. If we consume their GMO food, we cannot be either of these.

I like thinking that God's creation is taken care of, and we are the caretakers. This is a God-given responsibility we must all accept willingly and happily. What has been given to us is perfect: now that man is destroying creation with his scientific madness, let's make billions of points of view.

Original Organic Food

Organic is a labeling term that indicates that the food or other agricultural product has been produced through approved methods. These methods integrate cultural, biological, and mechanical practices that foster the cycling of resources, promote ecological balance, and conserve biodiversity. Synthetic fertilizers, sewage sludge, irradiation, and genetic engineering may not be used.

Organic and biodynamic food is natural food. It is grown in healthy soil with all the natural microbes and minerals. There are no pesticides or chemical fertilizers used. If we could stop and think for a minute about organic food, we would never buy nonorganic again. Our minds will play games with us about how non-organic food is too expensive, so we have no choice but to buy factory-farmed food. This is wrong.

Organic food keeps much longer, tastes really good, and is full of minerals and vitamins—saving hundreds of dollars on doctor's bills.

Most Italians have wonderful vegetable gardens in their backyards. They are usually natural and overflow with rich red tomatoes, basil, and greens. They also have as many fruit trees that will grow in their garden. The beauty of this "practice" is hard for the average person to behold—as they trudge off to the supermarket twice a week to spend all their hard-earned dollars on factory farm food that tastes like nothing and lasts a day in the fridge. It is "disgusting" how supermarkets do not control the labeling of their poisonous food and make huge profits from farmers, making the farmers poor and the consumer reluctant (because of high prices) to purchase something as basic as fresh fruit and vegetables. When did fresh food become so expensive, we can't afford it anymore?

The world is not like it once was. The internet keeps everyone busy, so busy: playing games, talking to loved ones, promoting one's obscurity, watching movies; keeping their minds busy inside the screen while the corporations are changing the world around them.

If nothing else, a balance is called for, especially one that empowers each individual to be their own personal god. To be your best, exercise your powers for the good, and be the hero you are watching every day on your screens.

Detox

Glyphosate and GMOs are poisons that can be eliminated by ceasing to eat them, which will make your body much better after a few months. If you have a chronic disease, you can speed up this process by doing a few detoxes. There are quite a few different ways to detox, and this is just a sampling of them.

Celery juicing is popular and can be a pretty easy way to clean out your system for three months. You will need to buy organic celery every couple of days. Get one bunch of celery, wash it, cut it up, and blend it with some pure water and drink it before breakfast.

Moringa is a very powerful herb. It is common in South East Asia. You use the leaves of the tree and can eat them fresh or drink the juiced leaves or mix the powdered leaves with water.

Lots of reverse osmosis water every day (take a mineral supplement) will help clean you out as well. Many people like to start a detox with a coffee enema. You dissolve some natural coffee in pure water and slowly pump it into your nose while lying on your side. Be ready for it to come out along with a lot of different-colored chemicals that were stuck in your intestines.

An alternative to coffee enemas (you can get detailed instructions on the internet) is to eat only fruit once a week and drink a lot of water. This creates a flood of water in your system that washes out your intestines.

Fasting one day a week is becoming popular. This helps your body eliminate waste, rebuild the immune system, and keep you young.

Some of the best detox foods are grapefruit, Brussels sprouts, berries, beets, chia seeds, nuts, and bone broth.

To detox your body, you need to eliminate all junk food and alcohol, drink lots of water, eat good detoxifying foods, drink organic vegetable juices, and try some detoxifying techniques like enemas, celery juice, more sleep, and moringa.

Chlorella and Cilantro together can help you detox.

There is lots of good information on the internet about detoxing; it is worth doing the research to find a system that suits you. Detoxing can be as simple as eradicating all junk from your diet for a few weeks and eating only organic fruit and vegetables, or more detailed using special herbal combinations or enemas, juicing, and fasting.

Wildfit

WildFit is an incredibly popular program. It helps people around the world change their eating habits in 90 days.

Decades of food marketing have taught us to view food as the go-to solution in every life situation. This way of thinking puts humans inside a food prison; it gives food the power to define and control our emotional and physical lives.

Almost all food marketing messages point toward highly processed foods that are making people sick, overweight, and nutritionally deprived. Doesn't reading that make you both angry and incredibly sad at the same time? If you're fed up with this dysfunctional approach to feeding ourselves, you're in the right place.

If you've tried everything but still haven't been able to release excess weight, you're in the right place.

If you're sick and tired of feeling powerless around certain foods and want to genuinely enjoy healthier foods (but aren't sure that's even possible!), you're in the right place.

If you have goals and dreams that would be so much easier to achieve if you had more energy, better sleep, and improved focus, you're in the right place.

Internet Resources

Some of the resources I use every week are NaturalNews, Dr. Axe, GreenMedInfo, and alternative-doctor youwillchangetheworld. These four people are extraordinary. They offer incredibly good information for free. One is a qualified scientist, another is a qualified doctor, and the other is a qualified chiropractor. They are real angels and are doing more good for the world than anyone else I know. They survive by selling their books and natural products. Natural News (the health ranger) has a science lab and tests everything for glyphosate. Dr. Axe has very detailed info sheets on all healing modalities, and Dr. Mumby's books are ahead of their time. Greenmedinfo's books are well researched and offer clear advice on many health problems.

My father was interested in natural healing long before anyone else. He had a great library of books, and he loved to help people with cancer by exhorting the values of organic carrot juice. I am a slow learner (to the value of natural healing) and wish I had read all his books when I was young. In many ways, I have kept his dream alive in a small way. I prefer to write about health rather than be a practitioner because every time I try to help someone who is sick, they don't believe a word I say—they are programmed to believe only doctors. I guess my father de-programmed me, so that was a good thing for me.

Please trust the professionals I have listed they will get you off to a wonderful start (some articles in Natural News are contributions which may not be 100% proven) and keep you running for a thousand miles.

Summary

This book is short and hopefully sweet. In all the ZEN series of books, I have kept them very short so that the most important information is quickly accessible and also to encourage your own journey into these different worlds without copying my words verbatim. They are a gentle but enthusiastic reminder to wake up, control your mind, which will control your life, and make your free will work for the good of yourself and everyone else. There has been research done by an Australian nurse, who asked all her dying patients about their lives and regrets, and their answers were deafeningly tragic. This is what she discovered.

1. I wish I'd had the courage to live a life true to myself, not the life others expected of me.

"This was the most common regret of all. When people realise that their life is almost over and look back clearly on it, it is easy to see how many dreams have gone unfulfilled. Most people had not honored even a half of their dreams and had to die knowing that it was due to choices they had made, or not made. Health brings a freedom very few realise until they no longer have it."

2. I wish I hadn't worked so hard.

"This came from every male patient that I nursed. They missed their children's youth and their partner's companionship. Women also spoke of this regret, but as most were from an older generation, many of the female patients had not been breadwinners. All of the men I nursed deeply regretted spending so much of their lives on the treadmill of a work existence."

3. I wish I'd had the courage to express my feelings.

"Many people suppressed their feelings in order to keep peace with others. As a result, they settled for a mediocre existence and never became who they were truly capable of becoming. Many developed illnesses relating to the bitterness and resentment they carried as a result."

4. I wish I had stayed in touch with my friends.

"Often they would not truly realise the full benefits of old friends until their dying weeks and it was not always possible to track them down. Many had become so caught up in their own lives that they had let golden friendships slip by over the years. There were many deep regrets about not giving friendships the time and effort that they deserved. Everyone misses their friends when they are dying."

5. I wish that I had let myself be happier.

"This is a surprisingly common one. Many did not realise until the end that happiness is a choice. They had stayed stuck in old patterns and habits. The so-called 'comfort' of familiarity overflowed into their emotions, as well as their physical lives. Fear of change had them pretending to others, and to their selves, that they were content, when deep within, they longed to laugh properly and have silliness in their life again."

What's your greatest regret so far, and what will you set out to achieve or change before you die?

I wish, I wish, I wish. Wishing is useless without action. Wishing without understanding that we have free will and will power is a temporary feeling of a life's experience that could have happened. Most people don't understand that a wish comes from the soul and is a quiet and beautiful plea to the personality to wake up and do what the soul wants. Alas, it is but a short window of opportunity before the negative and robotic mind keeps you going on some idea that came from your environment and not your heart. There is not much in your way when you get a message from your soul about "wishing you were healthier." Write it down, believe it, and cherish the wish until atoms of longing form into a concrete expression you can use every day to be happy and fulfilled.

Thank you for buying this small book. Lots of love and good luck with your new powerfully healthy and happy life.

Roditch

roditch@protonmail.com

·